I0092828

ULTIMATE GOUT CURE HANDBOOK: A 7 STEP RELIEF FORMULA TO STOP PAIN FROM GOUT INFLAMMATION IN ITS TRACKS

Gout Diagnosis, History, Science, Prevention and Natural Treatment Remedies

DAVID WHITEHEAD

Silk Publishing

© Copyright 2021 by Silk Publishing

All right reserved.

The work contained herein has been produced with the intent to provide relevant knowledge and information on the topic on the topic described in the title for entertainment purposes only. While the author has gone to every extent to furnish up to date and true information, no claims can be made as to its accuracy or validity as the author has made no claims to be an expert on this topic. Notwithstanding, the reader is asked to do their own research and consult any subject matter experts they deem necessary to ensure the quality and accuracy of the material presented herein.

This statement is legally binding as deemed by the Committee of Publishers Association and the American Bar Association for the territory of the United States. Other jurisdictions may apply their own legal statutes. Any reproduction, transmission, or copying of this material contained in this work without the express written consent of the copyright holder shall be deemed as a copyright violation as per the current legislation in force on the date of publishing and the subsequent time thereafter. All additional works derived from this material may be claimed by the holder of this copyright.

The data, depictions, events, descriptions, and all other information forthwith are considered to be true, fair, and accurate unless the work is expressly described as a work of fiction. Regardless of the nature of this work, the Publisher is exempt from any responsibility of actions taken by the reader in conjunction with this work. The Publisher acknowledges that the reader acts of their own accord and releases the author and Publisher of any responsibility for the observance of tips, advice, counsel, strategies, and techniques that may be offered in this volume.

CONTENTS

INTRODUCTION

An ounce of prevention is worth a pound of cure.

— BENJAMIN FRANKLIN

Thank you for purchasing *The Ultimate Gout Cure Handbook!* Perhaps you are looking to treat gout, or you know you might be at risk and are seeking to avoid it. Perhaps you are just curious. Whatever the reasons you are looking at this book, I hope that, after reading it, you will know what you need to do to beat gout. You will understand precisely what gout is, why you got it, and how to make sure you never get it again.

In the first section, we will look at the past, for just a moment, and learn what history has taught us on this painful condition. I'll make sure you know what made me want to write this in the first place, then we will learn all about making your body as inhospitable to gout as possible. By no coincidence whatsoever, almost all the diet and lifestyle changes recommended in fighting gout carry over to general health and well-being, too!

There are a lot of treatment options out there, and I am pleased you chose my book. I have tried to present the information in a clear and entertaining while being as concise as possible. I hope to give you the tools you need to enjoy all the foods and drinks you want without waking up in the morning with a throbbing, red big toe!

HONEYMOON'S OVER

MY PERSONAL STRUGGLE

I married my wife on August 15th, 2009, when we eloped to Hawaii. Risking the wrath of both her and my families, we took an extended weekend to Oahu, had a justice of the peace sign the certificate, and spent the whole rest of the weekend eating, drinking, and otherwise making the most of our tropical getaway. We were both closer to midlife than either of us cared to admit. When we got back to reality, I had a pain in my toe, and we just wrote it off as too much beachcombing.

However, as the years went by, it would happen again and again: a feeling like needles, hot needles with a burning sensation that can wake you up at night. Tingling, throbbing, and super sensitive, it almost feels like a raw wound. The affected area is visibly red, inflamed, and swells like a bruise. It wasn't until the third time it happened that I went to my doctor and diagnosed it as gout. He offered me a prescription, but at that point in my life, I was still fairly convinced of my invincibility and said I'd treat it on my own. He gave me a few stern warnings about returning if it got worse, how it can lead to debilitating arthritis, kidney stones, and joint damage if left too long.

Okay, Doc, I get the picture: if it comes back worse or doesn't go away, we'll see you.

As I dug into the topic, I began to see that it was no wonder my first episode had flared up while living it up beachside. There's a genetic component, too, so while my dad was never exactly forthcoming in talking about his medical stuff, I know he used to hobble around sometimes, for weeks at a time. Gout doesn't trouble him anymore, but he is taking medicine for it long-term, just another pill in the little pile he has to take every day. More than anything, this prompted me to start addressing the causes and cures with diet and exercise. I would do everything I could to treat gout myself instead of taking a pill for the rest of my life.

Gout *is* excruciating and not something I want to take chances on ever getting again.

Big Toe

I am your big toe. Now, let's be realistic here; while this whole new world of pain could be almost any joint in your body, it's usually me. I am the first hard turn our blood makes after leaving the heart. The Descending Aorta is 2.5 cm across, that's a few hairs shy of an inch, and it moves all the blood used by the lower body downward.

Between heartbeats and being pulled by gravity, our blood is positivity rushing toward our feet.

By the time this blood superhighway reaches your hips, the femoral artery is about 6.5 mm, a quarter of an inch now, where it courses down along your femur. Our blood keeps rushing earthward where it finally hits me, and if it doesn't immediately go back up in the opposite direction, it snarls and splits into the thousands of little tiny veins that help make me, and the rest of our foot, oh so sensitive.

Right about now, I am quite a bit swollen, tender, and red. I woke you up out of a dead sleep, throbbing and sore. Tender and inflamed, you think maybe you scraped me against some coral, stepped on some kind of stingy ocean thingy, or maybe sprained me walking funny in the cheap hotel flip-flops you had to buy because you forgot to pack some.

Nope.

As our blood loops around our entire circulatory system, making one complete lap in about one minute, it only makes sense that most of the jagged little bits would get hung up in me first: Your first significant cul-de-sac. Blood slows down, deposits what it's carrying every bit like a river dropping sediment along a bend.

All the strange foods you don't normally eat, and exotic drinks you don't usually drink, have collided inside your body. Those salts have piled up here, in me specifically, and now you have a disease. Very much in line with the origins of that word, Dis-Ease, you are not at ease, wincing when you walk or pokes curiously at the red, raised area along my edge. It hurts to walk, and it hurts to hold still. It hurts when I'm heated up or when you are stressed. Making me cold with a bag of frozen veggies chased the pain away a little bit, and that's what made you think I was just an injury and not a symptom of an actual internal malady.

In the meantime, the slightest breeze is enough to send even more pain shooting through your foot. Sure, in a week or so, I'll be back to my old self again, and since you are not scarfing down all-you-can-eat seafood and putting down a few more drinks than usual, I'll be pain-free for months, even a year.

But just you wait.

You're not getting any younger, and the very same factors which made me flare up into an angry red match head in Hawaii only lower their thresholds as you get older. Even now, as you tuck into a steak dinner, washed down with a beer after not getting enough water all day, I can feel the uric acid building up faster than it can be flushed. I can feel the needle-shaped salts stick together and clump to my arterial walls, only to get washed away before you are even aware it's happening. It happens again and again, and each time, less and less uric acid leaves your system.

2

GETTING TO KNOW GOUT: THE HISTORY

YOU ARE IN GOOD COMPANY

So, you have gout. Well, it turns out you are in good company- or at least illustrious. You may even see it called The Disease of Kings! For centuries gout was blamed on an idle lifestyle but it was later learned that the rich seemed to be the only ones getting it was because they were the only ones able to afford red meat and the other foods which trigger gout.

Henry the Eight famously suffered from gout, and with so many images of him holding a haunch of meat or tankard of ale, it is easy to see why; both those are classic triggers of a gout flare-up. While that particular monarch's penchant for decadence and indulgence is legendary, one didn't need to be an overeater or drink too much to get gout.

Isaac Newton was notoriously spare in his lifestyle. Newton was a devout Christian *and* an alchemist. Not only was he religiously devoted, but methodical in his observations, as well. His habits were positively lean compared to other men of wealth and influence in the day. Forever slender and never one to risk the ire of the Divine by displaying gluttony, Newton is an excellent example of getting gout by simply being unaware of what foods put you at risk and, possibly, not drinking enough water. Of course, that poor guy seemed to have died from drinking mercury, so I will make sure to avoid Alchemical cures involving 'quicksilver' in this book!

Benjamin Franklin was also afflicted, though it is a bit easier to imagine that celebrated lover-of-live may be over-doing it!

You might think that with lifestyle being a leading cause of gout, the number of sufferers would be dropping in our modern age, but such is not the case. More than 8 million people suffer from it, and those rates seem to be rising. Once thought to be an ailment of the idle and nobility, gout is now seen in athletes, young adults, and women, too. While good modern living has dramatically increased our quality and length of life, some of those foods can be detrimental when they get out of balance.

Many athletes performing at the top of their field have reported dealing with gout, including renowned New York Yankees and Toronto Blue jays southpaw David Wells. Basketball great Maurice Cheeks developed it once he began coaching after 15 seasons in the National Basketball Association. Note he didn't get it until he took a less physical roll. It's easy to remember to take care of yourself when you are sweating buckets all day, it seems. Australian professional soccer player Harry Kewell was only 27 and still playing when he was diagnosed with gout.

None of these high achievers are overweight, overfed, and at this level of performance, we have to assume, are doing everything they can to not only remain healthy but thrive and grow stronger.

The average person living in the industrialized world has access to enough food, so much of our diet is meat, and many do not drink enough water, while at the same time we struggle to maintain an active lifestyle.

GETTING TO KNOW GOUT: SCIENCE & MEDICINE

WHAT IS THE SCIENCE BEHIND GOUT?

HYPERURICEMIA IS GOUT

The medical term for an excess of Uric Acid in the blood is Hyperuricemia. Usually, uric acid forms in your blood when a substance called purine is broke down by digestion. When everything is working as it should, the uric acid formed in your blood is voided through your urine. Mostly unavoidable, purine is a naturally pervasive nutrient found in many foods your body needs. You use purines to make, among other things, DNA, RNA, and ATP, your genes, genetic protein production, and cellular energy, respectively. These are crucial to life itself, so cutting purines out altogether is not only tricky, but I'm not even sure you would want to.

In any case, breaking down purines creates uric acid, which your body can't deal with in high amounts and is typically excreted in your urine or passed through your intestines and into your stool. Ensuring your body has the time to regulate this salty acid is part of keeping your system in balance and is a large part of what we'll be talking about in this book.

Left untreated, it's the kidneys and liver which take the biggest hit, as those two organs filter and cleanse your blood. So even if screaming pain and the sight of angry, red lumps on your foot, joints, or even on your ears doesn't motivate you, at least let the dangers you open yourself up to if left untreated move you.

Across the entire population, gout afflicts approximately 5.9% of men but only 2% of women. More than half of all gout sufferers are men because women have a lower uric acid level in their blood. The female hormone estrogen flushes uric acid out more efficiently, making women less susceptible to this painful form of arthritis. If too much uric acid builds up in the blood, it forms Urates, and these salts crystallize and then get stuck along your arterial, wall causing gout.

Usually, one's first and primary gout flare-ups happen along the big toe. Although the painful red swelling can occur anywhere, it is almost always in the joints, particularly the wrists, ankles, fingers, and elbows. Taking the form of raised, red areas of burning, inflammation, fever, chills, body aches and a limited range of motion can all go along with a gout flare-up.

If left untreated long enough, the crystals pile up and form nodules called Tophi, which remain in the joint to disfigure the body even when they are not red and inflamed. As soon as the first flare-up, these clumps of crystals are already irritating their surrounding tissues and causing you pain. Gout is a form of arthritis, and the knobby, swollen joints that are synonymous with advanced arthritis will be familiar to someone with extreme, advanced gout, too.

With so much understood about how one gets gout, it may have been a surprise to learn in the prior section that gout cases, at least in the US, are on the rise. This increase is because of our aging population, national food preferences, and a lower general activity level overall. Recent strides in genetic medicine have identified a hereditary component to gout, as well. Changes to a specific gene affect the body's ability to release urate into the gut, and it is the accumulation of urate in the blood which causes gout. If left untreated, these inflamed, pink areas can turn into hard, crimson knobs of tophi, which are not only disfiguring but cause real, permanent damage to the joint.

You may recognize part of the word Urine in Urate, and you would be correct, as it is precisely the same process connecting the stomach, kidneys, and bladder. Gout, let go too long, leads directly to those excess urates crystallizing in other places within your body, leading to not just inflamed or disfigured joints, but kidney stones, kidney disease, and even heart disease. Increasingly it looks like gout left untreated can also lead to hypertension, diabetes, sleep apnea, and even depression

So if you have a parent with gout, you may want to sit up and pay a little extra attention. For that matter, if you are a sufferer and have children make sure they take the following advice to heart. Prevention, as ever, is a whole lot easier than cure, as you will see when we get to the business of avoidance and remediation below.

Luckily there are some warning signs to look for to determine just how at-risk you are, whether you fall into the "A Little, Sometimes" group or in the "None, Ever" group. A history of unexplained pain in joints, stiffness, had arthritic symptoms earlier in life, or a parent who suffers all indicate you should be looking to cut your uric acid levels. However, because there is a substantial genetic side to this disease, lifestyle alone may not be enough to combat its flare-ups.

SYMPTOMS

It is essential to know what to look for, both by realizing what puts you at risk for gout, and having an idea of what it is not. Because there is not only a tendency of some people to casually call any red inflammation on the foot gout, but there are also a few ailments that look like gout, as well.

BEYOND INFLAMMATION

Burning red joints might get all the attention, but sometimes a low fever, chills, body aches, and generalized pain can accompany a gout flare-up. As if that injury is not enough, there is further insult added by the fact that gout flare-ups seem to happen more at night, specifically while you are sleeping. Not a wake-up anyone wants. The theory is that the body's lower temperature at night, your lack of water intake while sleeping, and a nocturnal lowering of cortisol are to blame.

❧ 4 ❧

GETTING TO KNOW GOUT: TRIGGERS

DIET, AGE, OBESITY AND MORE

Now that we know how gout looks and feels, let's look at how to avoid it. All sorts of things can set off an episode of gout, but by taking the following into account, you can not only shorten the length of an attack but reduce the chances of getting another one. Eliminating or limiting these triggers is the point, after all, and by taking the following to heart (literally, in some cases!), you will experience far fewer complications than doing nothing. Indeed, as we just read, doing nothing is a literal road to ruin.

There is an essential genetic component, as well, so if you do not have easy access to your birth father's medical history, there are blood tests that can be run to check how fast you metabolize uric acid. Some studies place the hereditary factors in gout formation at more than fifty percent, so getting this information can be essential to forming a gout-friendly lifestyle.

DIET

Maybe the most classic cause of gout is too much of the wrong kinds of foods. While the casual, routine ingestion of certain things can trigger an episode of gout, usually one has one's first flare-up following an unusual amount of it.

When we talk about a gout-friendly diet, we begin looking at everything consumed, and as you will see below, most are part of a healthy lifestyle already. The following should be incorporated into your routine as quickly as possible because the foods you need to limit to beat gout also have been shown to lower cholesterol, blood pressure, and weight. Many kinds of seafood are as much of a trigger as red meat, though some of the right types of fish offer far too many other health benefits to cut out entirely, as we will read below.

AGE

Yes, as we mentioned above, the image we may have in our mind of a stooped-over, gout-afflicted senior citizen is at least partially true. The older one gets, the more likely you are to develop gout. Indeed, out of all the female gout sufferers out there, the vast majority are seniors, the drop in estrogen causing a subsequent rise in uric acid. People often miss the fact that men have estrogen, too, albeit at lower levels than women, and just like testosterone, it also tapers or falls away in one's golden years.

It is easy to see why gout is far more prevalent in seniors when you pair that drop in estrogen with the relative inactivity of retirement. On the positive side, senior citizens often already have some gout-busting tools at hand. Besides the careful diet elders typically adhere to, walking aids, and heating pads are usually more readily available.

OBESITY

Increasing your heart rate is a pretty fundamental part of flushing fluids through your body. The exertion of heightening your heart rate, breathing harder and flexing so many muscles forces everything through your body's many interconnected organs that much faster. Without regular increases of your metabolism like that, your entire body gets a little sludgy.

As a matter of general health, there are many reasons to cut extra pounds, and it looks like gout is another. As you read above, gout happens when uric acid crystallizes in the bloodstream and gets stuck along the vein's wall. Chunky build-up along the artery is far more likely with the walls of your veins covered in the waxy 'fatty lipids' of cholesterol. However, even with healthy cholesterol levels, a high Body Mass Index causes more uric acid salts. Chemistry in the blood itself fosters crystals easier, and so much salt builds up in the body that it can't flush fast enough, so it accumulates.

This biological reaction in an obese individual's blood creates the perfect environment for gout to form. Not only is one's production of uric acid increased, but there is a decreased renal excretion of urate in urine, too. This is all to say not only are you making more uric acid, but you cannot pass it as efficiently, either.

INCREASED USE OF DIURETIC MEDICINE

Diuretics are a type of medicine that makes you urinate all the time, which lowers the amount of fluid in your body, making it easier for those pesky uric acid crystals to form in your joints. Of course, any doctor who has prescribed diuretics has most likely warned you about making sure to keep your fluids up by drinking lots of water, and it is always good advice in general. Hydration has been a health buzz-word for a while now, and we can add "avoid gout" to the relatively long list under Water's Health Benefits.

However, this book aims to treat gout naturally, or at least as naturally as possible. So while I will go over the common prescriptions used to combat gout near the end of the book, we will be focusing below on remedies, treatments, and therapies you can use at home or at least after a quick trip out.

GETTING TO KNOW GOUT: IS IT ACTUALLY GOUT?

COMMONLY MISTAKEN WITH GOUT

Before we jump into treating gout, let's make sure we understand what Gout Is Not. While writing this book, several friends and family have come forward and asked, "Is this gout?" and, with relief, so far, I have not had to say, "Yeah, probably." Some people I talked to were either already taking preventive measures or already had a flare-up and were taking steps not to get one again. In the interests of being thorough and not barking up the wrong tree, let us go over the so-called 'gout mimics' you should be aware of before you begin to treat gout.

PSEUDOGOUT

If it burns like gout and looks like gout, is it gout? This popular cliche works when talking about gout and duck quacks because of CPP Crystal Deposition Disease and its uncanny resemblance to gout. CPP is Calcium Pyrophosphate, and just like the uric acid we talked about above, they are both an essential part of a healthy metabolism. Still, when out of balance, they can settle in the joints, crystallize and aggravate surrounding tissues, as well.

This one can be tough to differentiate between, sometimes requiring a doctor to physically take some of the fluid from the swollen area and check its crystalline structure under a microscope! The uric acid crystals are shaped like long sharp needles, while pseudogout forms as rhomboids, which are more like a squashed rectangle.

Without looking at the infected tissue microscopically, gout tends to first form on the big toe, and we see pseudogout initially show up in the wrists and knees. Pseudogout is sometimes mistaken for rheumatoid arthritis, but pseudogout is usually far more localized.

CELLULITIS (BACTERIAL INFECTION UNDER THE SKIN)

An infected joint caused by simple bacteria, cellulitis is quite severe. As a bacterial infection that has gotten under your skin, cellulitis can be quite terrible if it gets out of control and spreads. Horror stories of cellulitis left untreated include not just red, purple, or even black discoloration of the skin, but holes in the flesh, amputation and, even death! Luckily, this kind of infection can't get in without a cut or scrape, is generally identified as an infection right away. The speed with which cellulitis can spread makes it not something you ever want to second guess, so please make sure to seek medical help if you think you are looking at an infection.

RHEUMATOID & PSORIATIC ARTHRITIS

Another disorder that shows up as red, inflamed joints is Rheumatoid Arthritis. These symptoms accompany the same sort of red swelling that we see with gout. Unlike the raised red areas that gout creates, the cause of the red inflammation an RA sufferer experiences is unknown, and only about 25% of people with rheumatoid arthritis get them. Beyond blood tests and microscopic analysis of the nodules themselves, there is no easy way of differentiating the two. Since both show up quite commonly in people in their 70's and 80's, there are usually tests available if one's predisposition to one or the other is not already known.

Psoriatic arthritis is quite a bit easier to identify as separate from gout because of the so-called 'sausage finger' effect. The entire digit will swell up, and a feeling like it is inflating, or even like it is "going to pop," has been reported!

SEPTIC ARTHRITIS (INFECTED JOINT)

If only one joint is inflamed, it may be Septic Arthritis. Muddying the waters further both gout and Septic Arthritis can sometimes give you a fever and chills, as well as making you feel tired and lethargic. The body's natural response to an infection is to swell, but with gout, it is salts from inside the body, triggering the inflammation instead of a germ from outside.

STRESS FRACTURE

An injury usually causes stress fractures, so it is unlikely you will forget the incident which caused one. One may want to wave their hand and dismiss the pain from a break, but you have to think not only of the apparent stubs and impacts, but even taking an odd step up or down can do it, too. A broken toe or foot not healing right is not something you want to mess around with, so if you think that may be the case, it would be a good idea to try and get it x-rayed.

Now that we know we have gout and not one of its imitators, we can move on to the main event: let's beat gout!

Big Toe Continued

There is no doubt now I am clogging up with tiny needle-shaped crystals. Squishy cholesterol just hangs out along the wall and blocks stuff up, but the crystalline salts, which wedge in place along my veins, grate against my arterial walls causing pain and stiffness. The hard-edged barbs shred the vein lining where the excess uric acids have bunched up.

These tiny clusters of crystallized salts typically get dissolved away and flushed out, but if you just sit there doing nothing, they'll grow and grow until they begin to disfigure the skin and injure the bone! If left in a chronic state, they will not only expand, deforming and eventually causing permanent damage, but these little suckers can get caught up in the kidneys and cause kidney stones, or stuck in the liver causing liver disease, too. Ultimately, this toxic build-up can lead to heart disease or worse!

Lucky for us, you just started taking steps to flush those pesky tophi causing salts out of me and the rest of our parts. The right combination of foods and liquids, coupled with a bit more physical activity and less stress, have already begun to change the very acidity of the blood running through me. These changes unlock and loosen the crystalline formations that have formed and inhibit new ones from growing. Once, a tight cluster of jagged sabers, the crystallizing salts are now loosening up, breaking apart, and getting voided naturally.

❧ 6 ❧

GOUT PREVENTION

WHAT NOT TO EAT

There is so much made about what **not** to eat, if you wish to start with what you **can** eat, go ahead and skip ahead to chapter 7! If you do this, you have to bookmark this chapter and circle back to it when you begin menu planning. It can be discouraging to learn the Can Nots before the Cans, so I offer this option.

Maybe you do not have gout yet. Perhaps you had your first flare up and never want the feeling of thousands of red-hot needles poking the same place at once ever again. Whichever the case, it is a simple matter of choosing the right diet and maintaining at least the minimum of healthy lifestyles. The adage 'an ounce of prevention is worth a pound of cure' came to mind, and for a good reason.

By merely regulating the triggering foods' intake, one can enjoy some of them regularly, if not routinely. The exercise component is no more than the suggested physical activity recommended for anybody. Of course, if you are balking at the thought of Drinking More Water and A Little Exercise, you are probably plagued by more problems than gout already!

A gout-aware diet need not be only foods taken away. There are foods you can add to your diet that will help change your internal chemistry, making it less likely to accumulate those painful uric crystals. Before we explore the foods to favor, let us take a look at the foods to avoid.

THE MEATS

Your digestive system breaking down foods high in purine is what creates uric acid, and the body's inability to process high amounts of this acid is what causes gout. Limit or eliminate the purine, and your symptoms should go down that much quicker. Avoid these foods altogether, and you significantly reduce the likelihood of developing gout at all.

RED MEAT

It seems to be top of the list for gout avoidance. Lamb, beef, pork, most game animals like boar, hare, mutton, venison, and horse meat are all high in purines. These ruddy cuts are all included under the general term Red Meat and to be mini-mized if not cut out of your diet entirely. While pork does not generally fit the informal definition of red meat, as meat must be red or reddish-brown both before and after cooking to be considered red, pork is still termed red meat due to its nutritional content. These high purine meats get their red color from myoglobin in their blood, an oxygen-carrying molecule similar to the hemoglobin in our blood. Yes, I am afraid that bacon is off the table.

If you can enjoy red meat at all is going to depend on just how severe your tendency toward gout is. Because it's a matter of metabolism and nutrition, no two people will have the same gout severity.

SEAFOOD

Most seafood is high in purines. Especially true of mussels, shrimp, lobster, sardines, and anchovies, my introduction to gout was when my wife and I were honeymooning in Hawaii and eating all the foods either expensive or not even available back home.

Some fish discussed below are very low in purines and can be enjoyed in small amounts reasonably often. Again, however, this will depend on just how severely uric acid build-up affects you.

ORGAN MEAT

While not as popular as they once were, offal is still enjoyed by many. If one wishes to avoid gout, then it is advised one steers clear of foods such as liver, kidneys, heart, and tongue. "Sweetbread" is organ meats and can trigger a flare-up. While offal is exceptionally rich in B vitamins and minerals like magnesium and zinc, which are all great for combating gout, they are also unusually high in purines.

BEER & GRAIN BASED SPIRITS

You want to avoid or at least cut back on all alcoholic drinks during a flare-up and monitor exactly what kind and in what moderation you are drinking between episodes. Not only do grain-based spirits contain purines, but the sugars added or naturally occurring in many adult beverages are also an irritant, as you will read in the Sugar section below.

Vodka, whiskey, and beer are all high in purine and will trigger gout. While one may consider small servings of a gluten-free alternative, there are still purines in there, and differing needs of different levels of severity make this tough to recommend at all! One especially wants to avoid beers that are higher than average alcohol content (above six Alcohol By Volume), anything "barrel-aged" or "bottle conditioned" as these may still have living yeast consuming sugars.

SUGAR

Not just candies, sodas, and sweeteners but fruit and juice can be triggers for uric acid build-up as well. Fruit does have the benefit of some selections being high in Vitamin C, which is good for flushing uric acid. Many fruits, however, are too low in beneficial properties and should be avoided. Fear not; There are some fruits you can still enjoy, as we will read below.

The natural sugars in fruit are called fructose, and this can be extracted, refined, and is a ubiquitous sweetener in lots of foods. High-fructose corn syrup comes from corn and is super concentrated. Since the stuff is now known to be a common source of obesity, high-fructose corn syrup is not that difficult to avoid now as it used to be. Without processing it like that, the fructose in oranges is excellent: Vitamin C is good for equalizing the acidity of your blood, so in moderation, I recommend oranges and other citrus fruits. However, the fructose present in all fruits and many vegetables means your consumption of them has to be minimal.

While you want to limit all fruit severely, some you want to try and avoid altogether: Peaches, apples, pears, grapes, plums, and prunes all contain high purine levels and should never be on the menu. Honey, brown sugar, golden syrup, and palm sugar are all too high in fructose, and none offer enough benefit in keeping around.

CAFFEINE

Caffeine is a little different than all the other items on this list. There is a call for more research in several of the sources I was consulting since it seems that people who regularly drink two or more caffeinated beverages a day are not at risk of the stimulating substance causing a flare-up. However, in individuals who do not regularly drink caffeinated beverages or drink them less than twice a day, caffeine can sometimes contribute to an episode of gout within 24 hours!

The molecular structure of caffeine is similar to that of the common anti-gout medication Allopurinol. It's worth mentioning because the drug Allopurinol can trigger a flare-up in the first-time user, similar to caffeine's trigger on someone who doesn't usually drink it. This conflict between long-term versus short-term use, servings per day, and the varying levels in any given drink contributes to most taking caffeine off the menu entirely.

SALT

On the one hand, there is evidence that a high-salt diet can lower uric acid levels in the blood, but on the other, a high sodium diet can cause kidney stones, kidney disease, hypertension, and diabetes. Since all of those ailments can result from prolonged, untreated gout, it is a good idea to switch to a low sodium diet if you have not already.

❈ I ❈

SEVEN STEP GOUT
BUSTING FORMULA

So by now, you have concluded that something needs to be done about your gout, whether it is to combat an existing flare-up or ensure you do not ever suffer one. If we had a magic wand, this would be a one-step process because there is a single thing that causes gout: Too much uric acid in the blood builds up until it reaches the point that you can't move it through fast enough. The fundamental aim of this good is to make sure that doesn't happen.

Once you have your first gout flare-up, even if treatment begins immediately, it can take up to two years for the crystals to be wholly flushed away, and people may suffer flare-ups during that time. Taking the following steps will make sure that process is as pain-free and rapid as possible.

If you are already mindful of your diet and have at least a

little bit of physical activity in your lifestyle, then the adjustments you have to make will be slight. If you have managed to avoid setting a menu and getting your heart rate up for a few minutes a day, then it is time you began.

It can be darn tricky breaking bad habits or starting good ones. Our brain has strong pattern recognition, but this gets applied not just to patterns in our environment but also in our behavior and thoughts. Breaking the rhythm of your day-to-day routines can be jarring and make you feel uncomfortable, but this is simply a change; Growth. Many people will fail at making positive changes because of this initial discomfort, but if you can push through, it is a growing pain, and once it fades, you are more robust and in better health. It's as valid for making minor changes to diet and activity level as it is anything else.

A cool thing about the mind-body connection is just how quickly we can pick up a new habit. Between two weeks and two months is all it takes to change the brain and get to a New Normal. That is where you want to be: having identified these key points and incorporated them into your life, you are moving forward with a new skill set if you are thinking of gout at all.

Your Big Toe Conclusion

Healing and hale, I am flowing freely, our blood is at a healthy acidity, my veins are free of pointy little nodes, and my joints are freely bending with no pain. My irritated arterial walls have begun to heal, and I have not swollen up in weeks! I'm not burning or nearly as tender, though you will still be a little sore for a while. You will want to keep an eye, not only on me but the rest of your joints too.

I know I am gout-free now, but I want you to maintain these healthy habits: the food, the water, and the exercise together because there is no silver bullet for this beast. No one thing will keep gout away; we are prone to uric acid build-up, and there is no changing that fact. We have to adapt or suffer, again and again. You also need to remember not just to mind me but stay aware of any aches and pains throughout the rest of his body, too.

Gout is a herald. The pain and swelling a clarion call your body has trouble metabolizing uric acid. Assuming you are doing all these things, your system should have many defenses against many other complaints and disorders. We now know that kidney stones, cardio-vascular disease, and hypertension can all result from long-term gout, and thankfully all are also avoided by the same things we just learned.

❧ I ❧

COLD COMPRESS

In the order you may need them, let's start with easing the pain of a sudden flare-up. Cold applied to the gouty area will aid in reducing the swelling, and that should reduce the pain, as well.

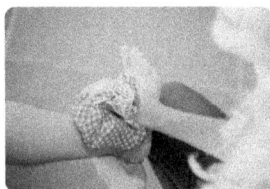

Upon the initial sign of gout symptoms, the first thing you need to do is get the inflammation down with a cold compress. No need for those fancy blue gel packs if you don't have one. A bag of frozen vegetables will work as long as the bag can conform to your foot. 20 to 30 minutes, and pain and swelling should subside.

On the other hand, in theory, overall cold weather should mean your cooler core temperature would make uric acid *less* soluble and more likely to hang around in the body and crystallize. But what happens is that more flare-ups occur in the spring and hot weather. The likelihood of an episode of gout occurring increases in places with a high temperature and low relative humidity; both conditions contribute independently.

. . .

While The Chills are a symptom of some gout flare-ups, this is not a natural effect of cold but accompanies the low fever and general unease that accompanies suffering gout. If you're dealing with other types of arthritis, you will want to use a heating pad.

RED GINGER

You can apply a compress of Red Ginger to an active gout flare-up for immediate relief. Taking two cloth napkins or small towels, shave two or three grams of ginger onto one of them, and lay the second. Bundle it up by the corners, and secure it with a rubber band or string. Soak this sachet in warm water, and then squeeze out the excess. Apply, still warm and moist, to the affected area for 30 to 45 minutes at a time. Some people like to make two and alternate between them every five minutes or so because you want them to be warm.

You should begin having fresh ginger in the house in any case because of the many dietary benefits we'll read about below.

ELEVATION

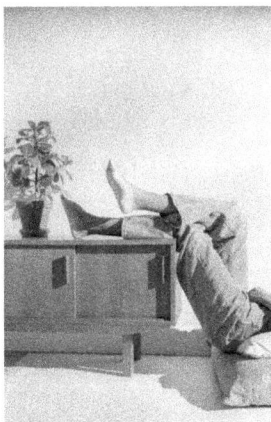

Propping the affected joint up during a flare-up is an excellent way to reduce pain. Depending on where it is, this may not always be possible. Even if the gout inflammation is in your ear, you should make an effort, at least, to be still and rest. If you can get the inflamed joint higher than your chest, it may help lessen the swelling, as well.

Keeping the afflicted joint elevated also lowers the blood pressure in the raised area. Putting it up will also increase drainage, helping the uric acid flush from your body faster.

If you have a crutch or cane, moving around will be ten times easier. A rod of any kind will help keep pressure off the joint and alleviate pain when you have to walk around. A single crutch is cheap and well worth hiding away in the back of a closet or otherwise keep on hand. Even if you do not have another episode of gout, there are all sorts of minor injuries you might want to have one around for.

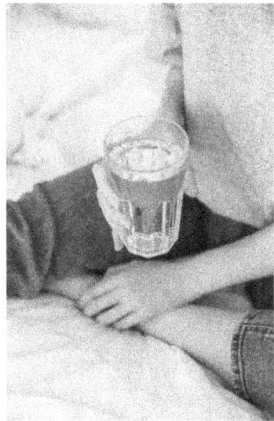

🏵 3 🏵
LIQUIDS

I am just going to go ahead get this one out of the way first. Fluids are so important, so primary to your overall health and well-being, that drinking enough water, at least staying hydrated, really cannot be over-emphasized. Without taking it to ridiculous extremes, one really can not get enough water. Fluid intake can include dietary moisture, and it keeps your kidneys and liver doing what they do best: flush your system. Nothing you eat, drink, or do will cleanse toxins and maintain your body's alkalinity in balance better than the organs of your body already dedicated to those jobs. Adequate hydration is even crucial for keeping your brain's synapses firing. It is just that important.

. . .

To keep your metabolism running smoothly for a typical adult trying to stem or stave off gout, about eight to sixteen cups of liquid per day is recommended, and more than *half* of that should be regular water. If tea, coffee, or any caffeinated beverage, you are well-advised to avoid it altogether.

However, there is a big difference between a regular drinker of caffeinated beverages and those who don't. We talked about cutting caffeine entirely, but if you regularly drink two or more servings of caffeinated beverages per day, the risk of it triggering a flare-up is minimal. In other words, if you are not usually drinking caffeinated drinks, the sudden spike in caffeine can cause an episode.

WATER

Can I just say it one more time for the sake of emphasis? Chances are, the first time you got gout, it was when you were neglecting your water intake. I was sweating, exercising, and drinking the wrong stuff for an extended weekend the first time it happened to me.

Be sure your area has good water, as some places are genuinely terrible. Increasingly, it is becoming clear that having too low acidity in your water is just as bad as having acid levels too high. Typically, you will already know if the area you are in has good water or bad, though it never hurts to double-check. Given the number of businesses dedicated to selling you water, filter systems, or dig wells, there is never a shortage of water quality information out there. Of course, you always have to be aware of whether the information you are receiving is an honest water quality analysis or a sales pitch.

If you do not already have one, get a filter for your tap water. A basic one should work, as you do not want to over-filter. You only need one f you are in a place with low-quality water, but you do not want to be wasting money on bottled. Everything being equal, as long as there is some mineral content, water is water as far as your body is concerned.

Minerality in water is highly beneficial so avoid "distilled" or "triple-filtered products." We are talking about pretty primary minerals here, so don't worry if your water is from Fiji, the fjords of Scandinavia, or wherever. A Ph balance close to seven and a slight mineral content is all you need to shop for as far as water is concerned.

Distilled water can leach minerals out of your body as you digest it, so make sure to avoid that. Even city-treated tap water has *some* dissolved solids in it, and distilling water removes those. Besides distilled water actively taking those elements out of your body on its way through, many people report distilled water tasting flat or otherwise not as tasty as usual. One doesn't typically think of water tasting like anything, though we all notice when it is bad.

MINERAL WATER

It can contain substances like magnesium, calcium, sodium, and zinc. Modern research suggests that some mineral waters can be a good source of those elements. We already know to avoid sodas and sweetened waters, but it looks like the benefits of natural sparkling water far outweigh any drawbacks, so drink up!

If you are on the go or otherwise can't get to a water source, then it is time for you to make use of a water bottle. While there are literal shelves of choices when you go shopping for one these days, you do not even need to spend money. One can usually look around and find a bottle with a cap or something to use as a canteen. Pick something you'd typically trash, and that's the Reuse part of Reduce, Reuse, Recycle. So now you are not only staying hydrated but keeping a little more plastic out of the landfill, too.

Once you find one that you like, you have to get into the habit of drinking from it. I avoid plastic ones because I hate the way it tastes and there is growing concern that some types of plastic can leach petrochemicals into the water and subsequently get consumed. Glass is known for not imparting any extra flavor to water, but metal is a better insulator for keeping things cold or warm. It doesn't matter to your kidneys, though, so just make sure you are drinking.

At first, you might find that water bottle coming home with you still filled up, but keep at it and, eventually, you'll find yourself filling it up at work, missing it when you forget it, and noticing a general better sense of well-being. Water is useful not only for gout but oral health, complexion, digestion, and more. Not getting enough fluids puts every system of your body under duress, bar none.

ALKALINE WATER

There is just not enough science to say, one way or another, just how beneficial Alkaline Water is. It seems like most credible studies on PH Adjusted Water indicate it is not worth the bother. The explanations I've read make sense: since your throat ends in your stomach and your stomach is full of acid anyway, the alkaline water you drink just gets re-acidified as soon as it hits your stomach. There are all sorts of claims are out there, and it's quite beyond our scope to say one way or another. I've never made it a part of my anti-gout menu. Again, though, water quality can differ from city to city, so a quick check of your local water's grade by a trusted independent source is always warranted, and usually just a few clicks, or a phone call, away.

SKIM & LOW-FAT MILK

In reasonable portions, you can enjoy skim and low-fat milk. While drinking a 6 to 8-ounce portion won't lower your uric acid levels, it does encourage your body to excrete more through your kidneys and urine. One study showed that while drinking soy milk elevated uric acid levels in the blood by as much as ten percent, they saw a 10% decrease in those levels from participants who drank the same amount of skim milk. The result of a substance in skim milk called Orotic Acid, the doctors who ran the study was quick to say more research was needed it know exactly how much is tolerable.

APPLE CIDER VINEGAR

While not directly related to gout, the only science-backed data I saw on Apple Cider Vinegar indicated it aids in weight loss and inflammation. Two things that gout sufferers are always looking to lessen. Be sure to dilute apple cider vinegar before drinking, as it is highly acidic on its own. Adding one tablespoon to a full glass of water is all it takes. Or, add oil and use it as a dressing on their salad. However, there are side-effects of too much ACV, so as always, start slowly or ask your health care provider.

JUICES

It is highly recommendable you always eat the whole fruit wherever possible, instead of just drinking the juice. Not only is this because makers will typically add sugars to a juice or filler fruits wrong for an anti-gout diet, but the fiber and other nutrients you get from the fruit are so beneficial. Home juicing is *a little* better, but if you are filtering or even taking out the pulp, you are taking away so many valuable parts you might as well eat it.

While I have already warned you to limit your fruits and juices, there are exceptions, so do not worry: there are still quite a few options open when you want a sweet drink. Indeed, some of these juices are even used regularly in a bid to lower your uric acid levels. Foods rich in Vitamin C, and even vitamin C enriched foods, disintegrate uric acid to flush from your body, but other compounds also aid in blood-acidity regulation. Let's take a look at those others first because Vitamin C has been encouraged for so long you may already have some oranges or Vitamin C tablets handy.

If you still want to drink fruit juice, get used to reading those labels, as there is every incentive for manufacturers to add sugar, high-fructose corn syrup, and other fruits than advertised. You will be doing more harm than good unless you avoid those additives and stick with 100% juice, or at least can confirm nothing on the label will spike uric acid levels.

CHERRY

Tart Cherry Juice has a significant impact on your uric acid levels. Drinking eight ounces a day for four weeks was seen to drop uric acid levels significantly, concentrate working as well as regular juice. Not just the juice but eating the cherries themselves seems to work, as well. One study found that by eating ten cherries a day, you could reduce gout flare-ups by as much as 35%, though we will explore eaten cherries and other foods below.

The red in cherries are compounds called Anthocyanins, which not only give cherries their color but actively lowers uric acid in your body. This same compound gives blueberries their blue color, though there have been no studies on blueberry juice and gout. Be sure not to get Golden Cherries or Sweet Cherries as these have more uric acid building fructoses than the Tart variety.

LEMON

Lemon juice is another exception to the No Juice rule. Similar to how the unique red chemical compounds in cherries actively neutralize uric acid in a gout sufferer's body, so do lemons and lemon juice. Citrus in lemon juice stimulates the pancreas to create Calcium Carbonate, which aids in the alkalization of your blood and urine.

It is interesting to note that while both these juices are high in sugar, and as we read above, sugary foods exacerbate gout, they contain chemicals active in working against the conditions in which gout thrives. While the sugars in these juices upset your body's uric acid levels to some degree, the compounds in tart cherry and lemon alter your body's PH Levels, even more, making the blood itself inhospitable to growing crystals. Couple these juices with increased water intake, and you'll be well on your way to never suffering another gout flare-up.

ORANGE

While the Vitamin C in orange juice does help lower uric acid levels, and the high fructose levels boost your risk, the extent to which vitamin C helps your body flush uric acid from your blood more than makes up for it. Orange juice is funny because it is rich in Vitamin C, which lowers uric acid levels, but it is also high in fructose, which spikes your blood acidity! It seems to be a question of balance and moderation. This teeter-totter between Good/Bad extends to all the fruit juices high in vitamin C, which we'll see below. Once again, it seems to be a matter of quantity and balance; not everybody processes Vitamin C and Uric Acid the same way. So if you have, for instance, a strong genetic predisposition (like your dad and grandad both suffered from gout), then you may just want to avoid OJ altogether.

It is important to remember I am talking about the juice itself, and if eating an orange a day, all signs point to yes, yes definitely one orange a day is worth the fructose. As I said at the top of the Fruit Juice section, you want to eat the fruit far more than you want to drink it, as far your body is concerned. However, it is worth repeating since fructose is a trigger. If you are currently flaring-up or extremely sensitive, then it will be best to avoid it.

PINEAPPLE AND TROPICAL FRUITS

Pineapple juice is an excellent source of vitamin C, and while it is sweet as all get out, those sugars are no match for all the vitamin C it contains. Kiwi and other exotic citruses are also funny in that "Good Vitamin C But High Fructose" way, so make sure you enjoy in moderation. I should be mindful of my audience because these fruits are only Exotic or Rare where I live. When we were honeymooning in Hawaii, I realized that so-called Exotic fruits are common-place. Different parts of the world, heck, even other parts of the United States, have a relatively dizzying array of fruits to pick.

I see Guava and Kiwi in mixes all the time, though, so you should know they are considered high enough in Vitamin C to be recommendable. Be aware that most juice mixes get pretty liberal with added sugars and types of fruit added, so if you want that fruit flavor, just eat the whole fruit if you can.

GRAPEFRUIT

While not everyone's favorite, the tart grapefruit is a darling of nutritionists everywhere. Like the other fruit options on this list, grapefruit is high in vitamin C but low in fructose. Vitamin C not only aids in flushing excess acid from the blood but is an anti-inflammatory as well, which is why you see it recommended to people living with arthritis all the time.

If you're taking certain medicines, you want to *avoid* grapefruit as there is a particular compound in grapefruit which stops your body from absorbing the medication. A well-established side effect, the label of your prescription will have warned you against grapefruit if that's the case. If you have concerns about how your medication might be affected by grapefruit, or are worried about anything in this book, ask a healthcare professional.

STRAWBERRY

As seen in the foods section below, I began seeing it as a juice quite frequently once I started looking for it. Since most blends are fortified with bogus sugars and gout-unfriendly fruits, if you manage to find 100% strawberry juice or it is mixed with other juices on this list, you should be okay. I have said it above, and I will say it below, when it comes to fruits- Eat It, Don't Drink It!

. . .

There is a compound in strawberries, Oxalate, which binds to minerals like calcium in the body and makes it harder to flush; This can cause a flare-up or make an existing episode worse. That is highly unusual, but if you are worried about a negative interaction, consult a health professional.

AMLA

New to me, this fruit is increasingly easy to find. Indeed, it may be more common than I realize. Sometimes Alma is called Indian Gooseberry due to its color and taste. Being rich in vitamin C makes it worthwhile when putting together an anti-gout diet. Though again, it is a juice, so you want to eat it if at all possible.

❦ 4 ❦

FOODS

Food! The entrée, the main event. While liquids and activity levels can wind up making a more considerable overall dent in body chemistry, this certainly is not the case if you're eating wrong. Remember, it was a diet rich in red meat, coupled with beer, grain-spirits, and general sloth, that led to gout historically being associated with the well-to-do. While it is certainly hard to say we all live like lords in this modern age, we maintain a rich diet compared to our ancestors.

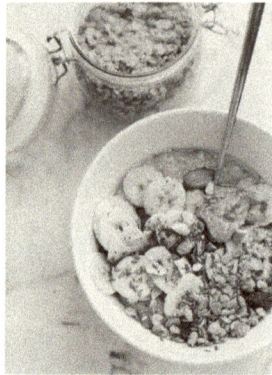

The ultimate goal is the decrease of uric acid levels in your blood, after all. We have to be mindful not just of purines, the breakdown of which inevitably generates uric acid, but of sugars and other gout stimulators, too. We have discussed the bans, so let's now focus on what we can enjoy.

CHICKEN

Generally low in purines, there are relatively high levels in some cuts of chicken. A moderate amount, so long as portions are limited to four to six-ounce portions per meal, you ought to be okay. A recommended Serving Size is usually about that, so by going low gout risk, we are also meeting the serving sizes prescribed for healthy living in general.

As you read in the chapter above, avoid all organ meats. I am afraid giblets, chicken liver, and all the rest are off the menu. Skinless chicken breast is the hands-down winner as far as cuts are concerned, so no more drumsticks for us. Recognize, though, how common a suggestion it is for skinless chicken breast in other aspects of healthy living.

FISH

Maybe seeing fish on here is a surprise after being warned off of seafood in general, but the oils and nutrients found in the right kind of fish are just what you need, as long as you avoid other purine-rich foods. Like fruit and other meats, there is a little purine in the following fishes, but as long as you observe your limits and remain aware of your portions, you can enjoy the fish below in moderation.

Salmon is a good source of Omega-3 Fatty Acid, long known

to reduce inflammation and lower bad fat in the blood, both things you want to do when treating gout.

Tuna and trout are two other fish packed full of enough good stuff to counteract the bad. We get into a bit of a grey area with fish as they do contain some purine, so it will differ a little on whether or not you can add a lot of fish to your menu or not.

Tilapia, flounder, whitefish, and sole are also options that you can include in your menu.

Even the fish we talked about above should be limited to two or three servings per week, in any case. As all fish seem to contain a little purine, if you are prone to uric acid build-up, you want to make sure your liver and kidneys have the time it needs to move it through your body.

NUTS

You can enjoy them; just don't go nuts. Some varieties contain more purines than others, but the low purine types are so full of essential goodness you can eat a few. Walnuts, almonds, flaxseed, and cashews are all excellent sources of protein and are also anti-inflammatories. Just a handful per day, though, as they do contain a little purine.

Peanut butter, as well as most nut butter, you may also enjoy. However, be aware as ever of the sugars added or extra refinements and adulterations and avoid them. You want just peanut butter, or whatever nut, as some of those sweetened ones have so much added sugar, it can cause a rise in uric acid.

CHEESE & DAIRY

If skim & low-fat milk is a good drink choice, where does that leave milk-based foods like cheese and yogurt? Cheese, yogurt, and cottage cheese are all low purine, and you can eat them freely. As long as you stick to the low-fat versions of those products, you can eat other dairy products, as it seems to be the fats in milk that bother those with gout as it is naturally low in purines.

EGGS

Low in purines and high in protein, eggs are a fine choice, though again, they do contain *some* purines. You will want to introduce them slowly as eggs can cause gout flare-ups in some people. Assuming egg is not one of your triggers, you can enjoy them however you like. Hard-boiled, you can eat them as is, but I like them sliced and on a salad. Just do not add salt. As has been mentioned, you should be monitoring salt intake in a significant way, in any case.

WHOLE GRAINS

Whole grain bread, quinoa, pasta, and rice are all recommended, though they contain a moderate amount of purine. The vitamins and fiber in whole grains more than makeup for the purine, though. The problem comes when you bleach or otherwise process these grains. The refinement process removes both bran and germ, the most nutrient-dense part of the food. Stick to whole, unprocessed grain and, of course, eat reasonable portions.

The Gluten-Free fad has given the general population the idea that these foods are bad for you. Study after study finds that only about 1% of people are celiacs or allergic, however. I know a few people who claim gluten-sensitivity, though, so it might be something you want to monitor.

It looks like what is happening is that people who cut gluten from their diet also began eating smarter in general, living healthier. A little bit like a gout-free diet, the gluten-free diet requires a change to every meal. It forces you to rethink everything you put in your mouth. Of course, when making significant dietary changes, you will also cut fat, excess sugar and eat smaller portions. Who wouldn't feel better all-around doing all those things?

POTATOES

Following right up on whole grains, the so-called 'starchy carbohydrates' includes this staple as well. If you think the potato is bland, then I would like to challenge that idea. The famous "1,001 Ways to Cook a Spud" might be cut back to a few hundred by the time you remove the bad-for-gout recipes. The humble tater can be your best friend, however, being low in purines and fructose. You will want to avoid sweet potatoes, though, as they contain Oxalates leading to kidney stones if eaten enough. As we now know, anything that is a contributor to kidney stones can be a trigger for a gout flare-up.

SOUP

With such a broad category as soup, you have to be careful, but the rule is: as long as the soup doesn't contain the triggering foods, you will be fine. Make sure it meat broth or meat extract-free. No seafood or beer broths or ingredients from the Trigger Foods list, either. That is why I put the foods to avoid before the foods to enjoy: this information is foundational. Any food I mention down here, with a variety or type that we said to avoid above, needs to be cut.

That said, there are tons and tons of excellent gout-friendly soup recipes out there, as most all of the low-purine foods go very well in a soup.

GINGER

Eat it, drink it, just get it. The ginger benefits are so wide-ranging I have begun to seek it out in restaurants, teas, and my home cooking. You will find I included ginger as a supplement below, as well. Exceeding four grams a day can cause disorders, so like anything that has a strong effect on the body, you do not want to overdo it.

Even using ginger topically has been shown to alleviate pain and swelling, as mentioned above. We keep a root of the stuff in our fridge as a matter of habit, as it can be grated or diced into lots of foods for a little added flavor.

CELERY

Long loved for its health benefits, celery is not only an anti-inflammatory but a no-sugar food, as well. I don't mean low-sugar; I mean no sugar. I laughed a little when I read that eating a stalk of celery burns more calories than you get from it, making it one of the only foods that cost more calories to eat than it gives you! Not a net-loss, however, because the stuff is packed full of vitamins and nutrients. If you are not fond of the flavor, there are other options.

Celery Seed is even more nutritious than celery and can be used as a topping or put into capsules. Once I began looking for it, I started seeing it as an extract, too! These methods are great for bypassing an unpleasant taste but still benefiting from the plant.

TURMERIC, GARLIC, AND ROSEMARY

Spices and herbs, I have included these plants in the supplements section below as well. Anything that you can find with bonafide anti-inflammatory properties will be your friend in combating flare-ups, as long as it low or no purines.

Turmeric is also a popular antioxidant, making it relatively easy to find, either in foods or supplements. It is not just the chemistry that makes it good for your blood's acidity, the actual shape of turmeric has a curative aspect. The nanoparticles are even more effective at helping rid uric acid from the blood than an anti-inflammatory agent alone.

5

ACTIVITY

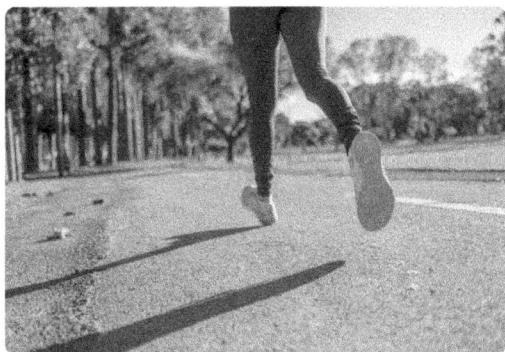

You will be wanting to look at getting your heart rate up but only once your flare-up goes down! During a gout attack, the throbbing and shooting intensity of even low-level activity can be overwhelming, so this advice should be easy to follow. Even if you can "push through the pain" or even find yourself needing to try, you want to rest the joint. Remember, the cause of gout is millions of tiny lances of uric acid crystal clustered together, so forcing the affected area to move can not only prolong a gout flare-up but will increase pain.

Once the flare-up has subsided, however, you need to get up and move again. If you are new to exercise, then start small. Walks, a little swimming, low-impact calisthenics, or any increase to your heart rate will give you the heart-health you need. In the beginning, you always want to choose low impact anyway. If you are unsure what is meant by Low Impact, it is precisely that: something non-jarring that does not place impact stress, intense cardiovascular jumps, or other shocks to your body.

If you are already engaged in regular physical activities, keep them up. Just mind your liquids and bad foods, yet another example of an excellent gout-free lifestyle causing a chain-reaction toward better health in general. As for gout, the increase in respiration is what pushes your blood through the cleansing organs faster, and the more rapid heart rate physically agitates the crystals where they are sticking along your arterial wall.

❧ 6 ❧

NO STRESS LOW STRESS

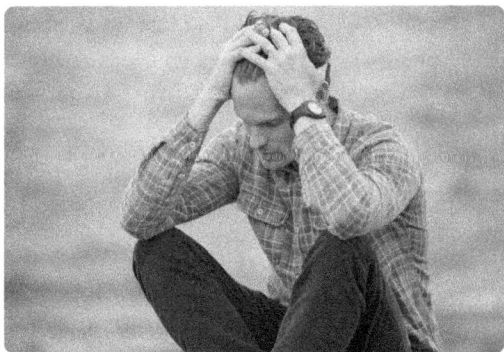

Under stress, the body loses its ability to defend itself. We have known this a long time, and it's an experience any adult has had. You get over-worked, not enough sleep, and otherwise keep your body under duress, and you get sick. The cause is even more direct with gout, as stress inhibits Pantothenic Acid from being formed, and the body uses this good acid to remove uric acid.

Listen to music, read a book or watch a show. Nothing too

gripping, mind you! Getting a bit of wearable technology which monitors heart rate is not a bad idea if you work in a busy environment or are prone to anxiety. Make sure you find one that is comfortable so you can wear it to sleep. Most of those things can track not only how long you sleep but what kind of sleep you are getting.

Some people prone to gout may get a little worried about going to bed for the night, as that is when gout flare-ups occur more frequently. You can not allow that to get in the way of a solid eight hours, though. Because sleep is when your body heals the most, getting as solid of eight hours as possible is crucial. Like water and exercise, it is an element of gout-friendly living which increases your entire constitution. If you have insomnia or troubled sleep, it is worth tackling as seriously as gout.

If you are exercising regularly already but still have trouble going to sleep, then you may want to try a few relaxation exercises or self-hypnosis. Even moderate activity should leave the body tired and ready to sleep. If you find your mind still keeping you awake, those tricks and methods can help calm you down for solid, uninterrupted sleep.

Reducing stress has far-ranging effects on general well-being, as well. Science has long since identified high-blood pressure, depression, cardiovascular disease, arrhythmia, and more as results from chronic stress. Of course, it is virtually impos-sible to remove all stressors from your life. You can begin avoiding unnecessary aggravation more and changing your attitude once you are aware of them. Permit yourself to lay pesky ideas your brain sometimes gnaws on to rest. Easier said than done, I know! A good rule of thumb is: if you cannot do anything about something *right now,* you should be able to let it go. I know there are entire industries based around doing just that, but with even a little bit of reflection and practice, it is incredible just how much control you have over what is going through your head.

SUPPLEMENTS AND MEDICINE

DRUGS

Never take aspirin for the pain of gout flare-up, as that can worsen it! There is a high-dose level at which aspirin increases uric acid excretion, but the breakpoint between the two will differ from person to person. So unless you are using aspirin under a medical medical professional's advice, skip the aspirin and use one of the following. While the whole point is curing gout as naturally as possible, many of us at least use a little of the everyday, over-the-counter medicines on occasion. In the case of a nasty flare-up, it can be helpful to know what one can use.

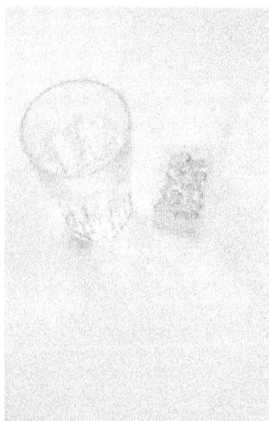

. . .

Ibuprofen, sold under the name Advil, among others, might be suggested to relieve aches and pains. Usually, if you have any problems with Ibuprofen, you will know by now, but as will any new medicine, if you have never taken it, please consult a health professional.

Naproxen, sold under the name Aleve for instance, is another nonsteroidal anti-inflammatory. Recommend for rheumatoid arthritis, osteoarthritis, and other joint diseases as well.

GINGER

Ginger is another famous folk remedy for swelling that is backed up by clinical research. Besides anti-inflammatory properties, ginger is good for digestive health, cardiovascular disorders, vomiting, and even some cancer types! Ginger is also a noted antioxidant with antimicrobial properties. It will not only ease some of the symptoms of aging but fight infectious diseases as well.

As I mentioned above, making a compress out of Red Ginger can offer immediate relief to an active flare-up. Being effective both topically and orally makes ginger one of my favorite remedies, as it not only tastes delicious but can be rubbed directly on a sore spot.

TURMERIC

As mentioned in the foods section above, turmeric is fantastic. Just like ginger, you may want to add it to everything, as well! While it works great as a spice, some may not like its taste, so you can always get it in capsules. While never a good as fresh or whole, as long as the pill contains unrefined turmeric, it is good. It turns out the turmeric nanoparticle, which is the technical word for the teeny-tiny little bits of the stuff, actually does as much good for you as the chemistry of the turmeric itself!

FISH OIL

Fish Oil can be an excellent option if you want the health benefits of the Omega 3's and other helpful elements but none of the purines. As long as you can be sure it is highly purified and rigorously distilled, good fish oil can give you all the benefits of fish with none of the uric acid causing purines of the fish itself.

Many fish oils on the market are impure, and I have seen information about much of the fish oil on the shelf being spoiled before it gets sold. In the case of some dishonest makers, it may not even be fish oil at all! The FDA classifies fish oil as a Food and not a Medicine; this means there is relatively less oversight. I am afraid it is buyer beware, which is to say a little research on the brands you are looking at might be a good idea.

BROMELAIN

Found in Pineapple, this complex molecule has anti-inflammatory properties and has only just begun to get clinical attention. Bromelain is also used to combat other forms of arthritis and sinusitis, and other inflammatory ailments.

PRESCRIPTIONS

Since the following are all medications requiring a prescription, I hesitated to include them at all. Doubly so this being more concerned with doing it yourself or otherwise using home remedies as much as possible. The names of the significant gout scripts are always good to know, though, as not all countries have the same laws surrounding the same medicines, so who knows. Maybe a few of these are over-the-counter where you live. None of these should be used outside a medical professional's advice, in any case, as these represent the most potent possible drugs.

NSAIDS

These nonsteroidal anti-inflammatories include Celecoxib, indomethacin, meloxicam and, sulindac. Many of these stimulate a gout flare-up initially before the body readjusts, and they begin working, so again, consult a professional.

The prescription steroid Colchicine controls inflammation, and you should continue to do so if you are already taking it.

The list of other medications available by prescription that have been effective at treating gout includes Allopurinal, Canakinumab, Probenecid, and Lesinurad. These medicines come with a strong warning, so again, I cannot point you in their direction so much as I am being thorough and bringing your attention to the fact that these options exist. Should you find yourself wanting to use a medicine, in addition to the advice given above, the prescribing physician will most likely also recommend all that I just went over, anyway!

AFTERWORD

Thank you for taking the time to read what I've laid out here, and I hope you've already begun to take a few of these steps. Beating gout yourself is possible. You just have to be systematic, tackling your routine from the top-down. The right foods for breakfast, lunch & dinner, sleeping, and stress are all equally important. One can not ignore one without weakening your whole defense.

I hope it was informative and that I could keep you engaged as I regaled you with what I learned on my journey to gout-free living. While it is no doubt you had your first gout flare-up from overeating the wrong kinds of foods, and drastic changes can feel so jarring, you just have to trust that you are creating a New Normal. The mind adjusts, and a strange new activity or food soon becomes a habit, and eventually, *not* doing these things will feel just as odd as doing them once did.

The next step is to take these lifestyle changes and make them permanent. Almost nothing I've suggested treats gout alone. Almost all of the advice is in keeping with all we know of general wellness. By choice, I've steered clear of the term 'Holistic' since there are quite a bit of scam out there answering to that name. That word has merit, not just in the spirit of using nature's remedies but also the root word 'whole.' Since the entire body benefits from every suggestion above, there is quite simply no reason not to follow this guidance. Of course, if you found this book helpful, entertaining, or otherwise engaging in any way, a positive review on Amazon is always appreciated!

GLOSSARY

HYPERURICEMIA

The medical term for too much uric acid in the blood.

PURINE

A naturally occurring crystalline compound found in many foods and drinks.

TOPHI

Clusters of crystallized uric acid which are built up over many attacks.

URATE

The salty crystal formed of excess uric acid.

URIC ACID

Also called Serum Uric Acid, this salt is formed by the break-down of Purine in your body.

www.ingramcontent.com/pod-product-compliance
Lightning Source LLC
Chambersburg PA
CBHW022105020426
42335CB00012B/840

* 9 7 8 1 9 8 9 9 7 1 2 0 8 *